# Zero Sugar Stevia Cookbook

Delicious Sugar-Free Stevia Recipes That
Are Naturally Sweet

BY: Stephanie Sharp

Copyright © 2019 by Stephanie Sharp

# License Notes

**Copyright 2019 by Stephanie Sharp All rights reserved.**

No part of this Book may be transmitted or reproduced into any format for any means without the proper permission of the Author. This includes electronic or mechanical methods, photocopying or printing.

The Reader assumes all risk when following any of the guidelines or ideas written as they are purely suggestion and for informational purposes. The Author has taken every precaution to ensure accuracy of the work but bears no responsibility if damages occur due to a misinterpretation of suggestions.

wwwwwwwwwwwwwwwwwwwwwwwwww

# Table of Contents

Introduction .................................................................... 6

   Guava Passion Drink ................................................. 8

   Grapefruit Fat Bomb ................................................ 10

   Jello Mug Cake ......................................................... 12

   Stevia Syrup .............................................................. 14

   Strawberry Shake ..................................................... 16

   French Tea Cream .................................................... 18

   Stevia Chocolate Mug Cake ..................................... 20

   Macedoine Frappe ................................................... 22

   Sticky Buffalo Chicken Tenders .............................. 24

   Prunes in Tea Jelly ................................................... 26

   Admiral Punch .......................................................... 29

   Scrambled Eggs with Cranberries ........................... 32

   Strawberry Lemon Juice .......................................... 34

Strawberry Cheesecake Mousse ................................................. 36

Tea Julep ................................................................................. 38

Chia Pudding .......................................................................... 40

Apple Cheddar Waffles ........................................................... 42

Grape Tea Punch .................................................................... 45

Mug Birthday Cake ................................................................. 47

June Plum Drink ..................................................................... 50

Yellow Bird Stevia Cocktail ................................................... 52

Chocolate Berry Cheesecake .................................................. 54

Zucchini and Carrot Noodles with Tomato Sauce ......... 58

Simple Tapioca Pudding ........................................................ 61

Delicious Banana Nut Oatmeal .............................................. 63

Tea Ice Cream ......................................................................... 65

Rum Punch .............................................................................. 67

Mug Banana Bread .................................................................. 69

Instant Pot Blueberry Oatmeal ............................................... 71

Avocado Salsa Zoodles ................................................... 73

Conclusion ........................................................................ 76

About the Author ............................................................. 77

Author's Afterthoughts ..................................................... 78

# Introduction

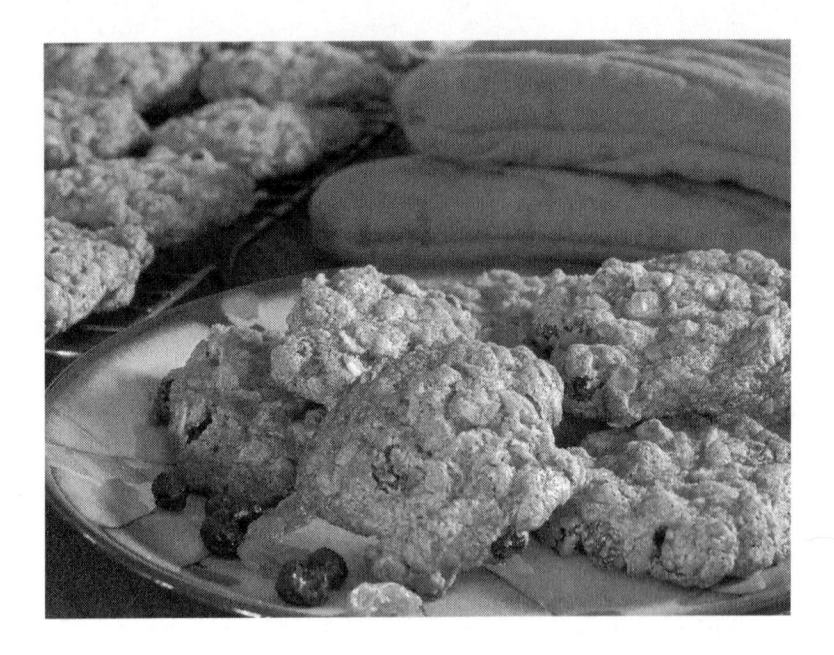

Thank you for snatching a copy of this Zero Sugar Stevia Cookbook. Everybody knows that a lot of sugar is detrimental to us as individuals. Sugar contributes to more than 70 illnesses—many of them dangerous and some incurable. I will give you some examples:

Obesity: All the carbs that we get from sugary foods are not simply discarded; they are stored, as fat, everywhere in the body like criminal loot. This is the real source of obesity.

Leads to addiction: An extremely high blood sugar level causes the body to overcompensate and release a flood of enzymes that will clean up the sugar. Then the blood's sugar level gets too low and triggers a series of symptoms such as headaches, light-headedness, among others that normally means a need to ingest more sugar. This causes a vicious cycle of constant desire for sweet food.

It leads to a malfunction of the immune system.

Contributes to Teeth Cavities: During the interaction of sugar and bacteria in the mouth, an acid is formed, which destroys the layer of hard protection for the tooth.

Also, it violates the process of metabolism in the body which contributes to the development of diabetes.

It contributes to the early appearance of wrinkles, as it changes the structure of collagen and reduces the elasticity of tissues.

Despite the evil effects of sugar, there are still value to adding taste to both savory foods and desserts. This Zero Sugar Stevia Cookbook will help you do just that. Here you will find 30 simple, proven and straightforward stevia recipes for delicious savory meals, desserts and juices.

# Guava Passion Drink

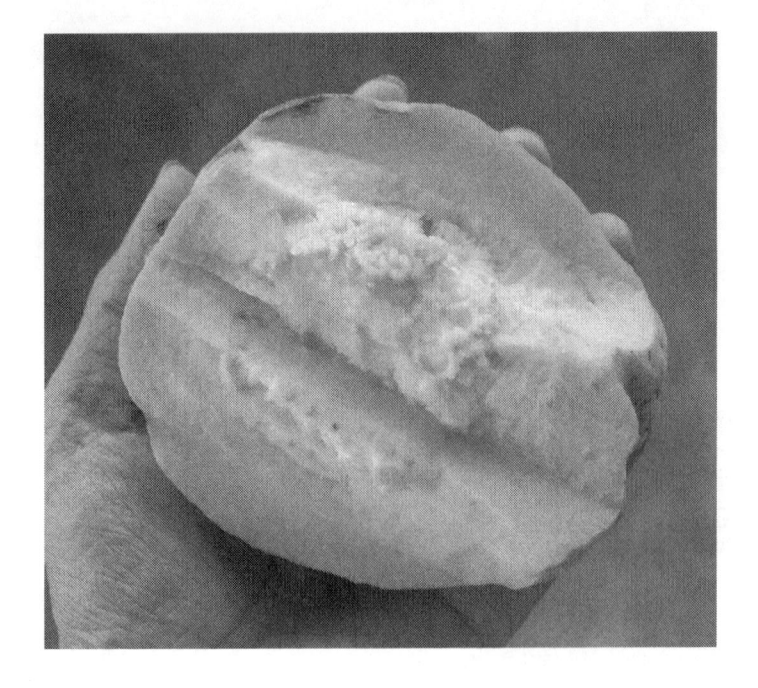

This is rich in vitamin C and makes an interesting drink.

**Serves:** 6

**Time:** 15 minutes

## Ingredients:

- 6 whole guavas
- 3 passion fruit
- 1 oz. lime juice
- 4 cups water
- 6 tbsp. raw stevia

## Directions:

1. Wash guava and passion fruit.

2. Dice guava and place in a container.

3. Cut passion fruit in two and remove pulp from inside. Place pulp in container with guava.

4. Set in your blender and process until smooth.

5. Strain and serve with cubed ice.

# Grapefruit Fat Bomb

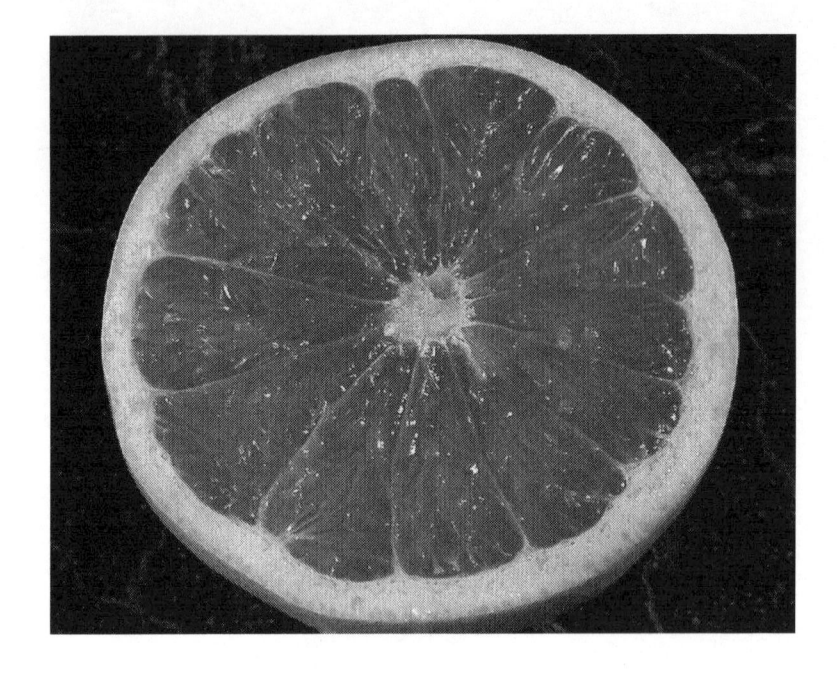

Here is a fat bomb recipe that you will never forget.

**Serves:** 4

**Time:** 2hrs. 10 mins.

**Ingredients:**

- ½ grapefruit
- 4 ounces cream cheese, at room temperature
- 2 ounces butter, at room temperature
- 2 teaspoons Stevia
- Pinch pink salt

**Description:**

1. Zest the grapefruit half with a very fine grater into a small bowl. Squeeze the juice from the grapefruit half into the bowl with the zest.

2. In a medium bowl, combine the cream cheese and butter. Add the sweetener, grapefruit zest and juice, and pink salt. Using a hand mixer, beat until fully combined.

3. Spoon the mixture into the fat bomb molds.

4. Freeze for at least 2 hours, unmold, and eat! Keep extras in your freezer in a zip-top bag so you and your loved ones can have them anytime you are craving a sweet treat. They will keep in the freezer for up to 3 months.

# Jello Mug Cake

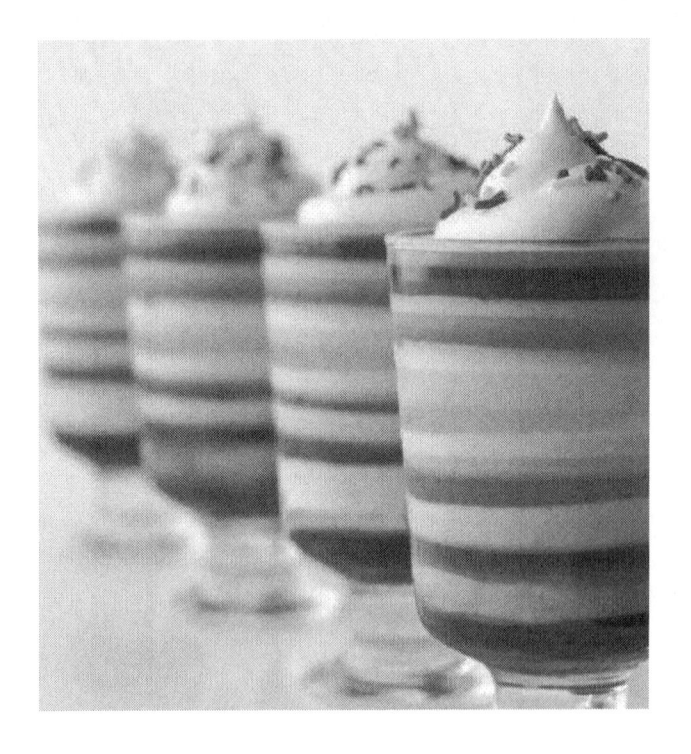

Try this tasty Jello Mug Cake and I guarantee it will leave you craving.

**Serves:** 1

**Time:** 15 minutes

**Ingredients:**

- Vanilla cake mix (1/3 cup)
- Jello (1 tbsp, strawberry)
- Oil (2 tsp)
- Water (1 tbsp)
- Egg white (1)
- Glaze
- Stevia (2 tbsp, powdered)
- Jello (1/2 tsp)

**Directions:**

1. Add the vanilla cake mix and 1 tablespoon jello mix into a mug. Add the oil, egg white and water, and whisk very well. Microwave for 2 minutes on high.

2. While the cake is cooking, add the powdered stevia and ½ teaspoon Jello to a plastic sandwich bag. Add some water and knead the bag to form a glaze. Cut a slit in the corner of the bag and drizzle over warm cake.

# Stevia Syrup

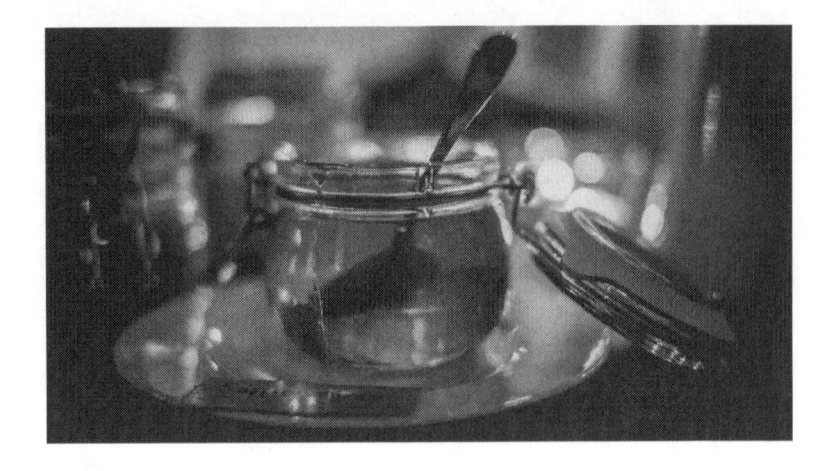

A nice stevia free base ingredient for liqueurs, and other mixtures.

**Yields:** 12 fl. oz.

**Time:** 15 minutes

**Ingredients:**

- ¼ cup stevia
- 2 cups water

**Directions:**

1. Combine ingredients in a saucepan on low heat, cooking until thick.

2. Pour in container. Use for lemonade and other mixtures.

# Strawberry Shake

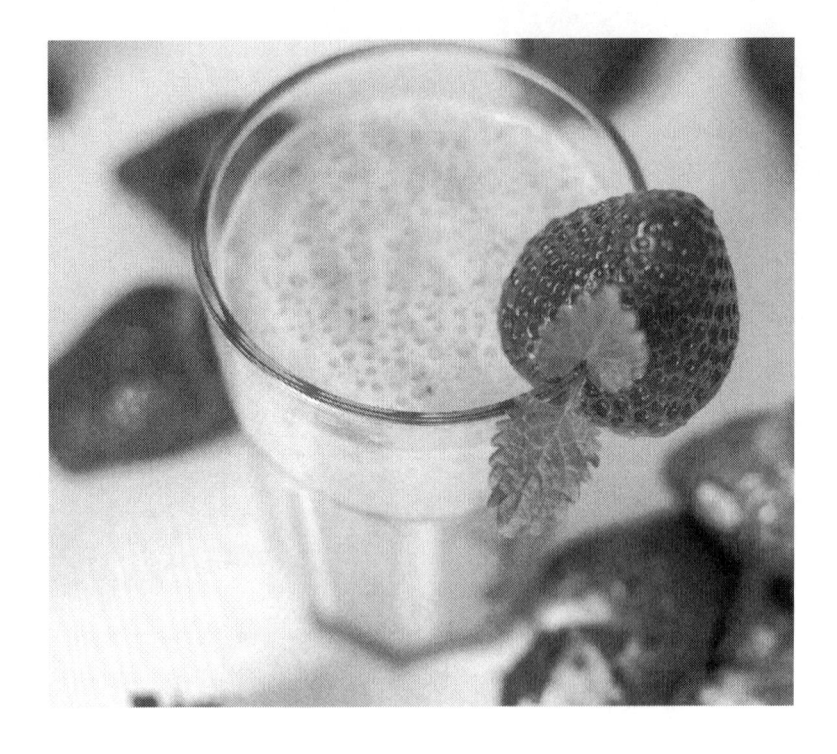

This delicious shake would be perfect for a hot summer day.

**Serves:** 2

**Time:** 1o mins

**Ingredients:**

- ¾ cup heavy (whipping) cream
- 2 ounces cream cheese, at room temperature
- 1 tablespoon Stevia
- strawberries, 6, sliced
- ice, 6 cubes

**Directions:**

1. Add all your ingredients to your blender then process until smooth.

2. Divide into two tall glasses and serve.

# French Tea Cream

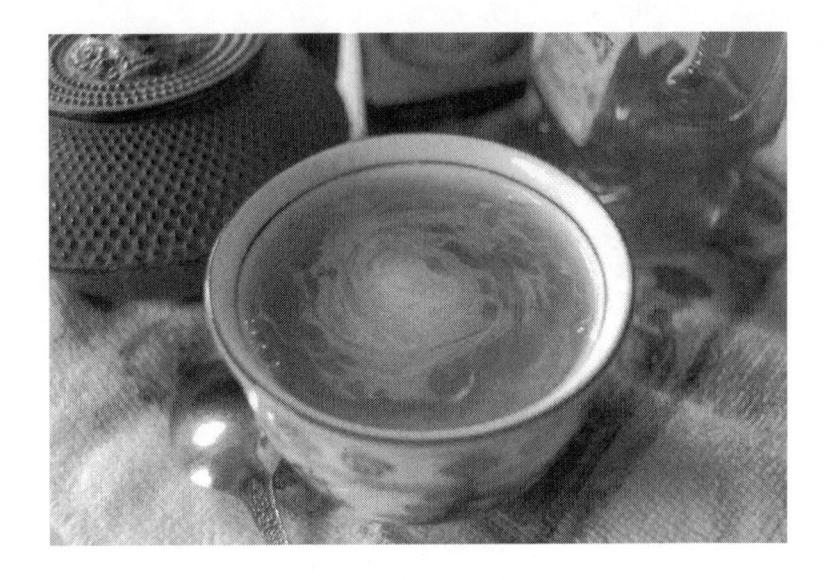

This dessert has a few steps but is still tasty.

**Serves:** 4

**Time:** 30 mins.

**Ingredients:**

- 1 quart of cream
- 1 tablespoon of loose tea (or 3 tea bags)
- eggs
- tablespoons of stevia
- 1 package of gelatin
- 1 cup of cold water
- whipped cream (optional)

**Directions:**

1 Scald 1 quart of cream. Switch off the heat and add a tablespoon of loose tea. Cover for about 6 minutes and strain tea.

2 Return to heat in a double boiler and add 5 eggs and 5 tablespoons of stevia which have been beaten together.

3 Stir until as thick as custard. Switch off the heat then add your gelatin solution (a box of gelatin diluted in a cup of cold water).

4 Stir until dissolved. Strain and set until firm.

5 Serve with whipped cream.

# Stevia Chocolate Mug Cake

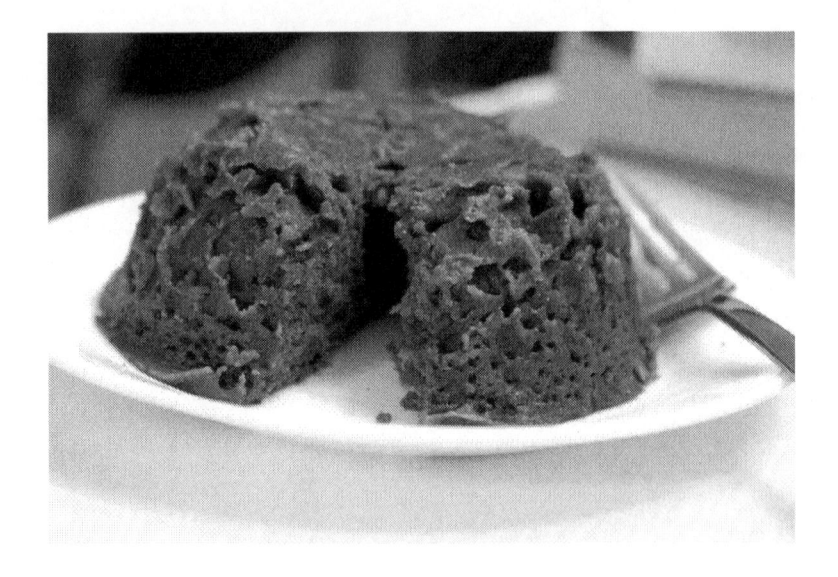

Try this sweet, homemade and delicious Company's Coming Chocolate Mug Cakes, a fitting desert for any occasion.

**Serves:** 8

**Time:** 5 mins

**Ingredients:**

- Devil's food cake mix (1 box)
- Chocolate instant pudding mix (1 package)
- Chocolate chips (1 handful, mini)
- Egg white (1)
- Oil (1 tbsp)
- Water (1 tbsp)
- Glaze mix
- Stevia (1/3 cup, powdered)
- Cocoa powder (1 ½ tsp)

**Directions:**

1. Grease a coffee mug with cooking spray and empty the cake mix into mug then add the egg white, oil, and water.

2. Blend with fork until well smooth and microwave for approximately 2 minutes.

3. While cake is microwaving, add water to the powdered stevia and cocoa powder in a sandwich bag.

4. After removing the cake from microwave, cut slit in sandwich bag and squeeze glaze onto the warm cake. Top with chocolate chips. Serve immediately.

# Macedoine Frappe

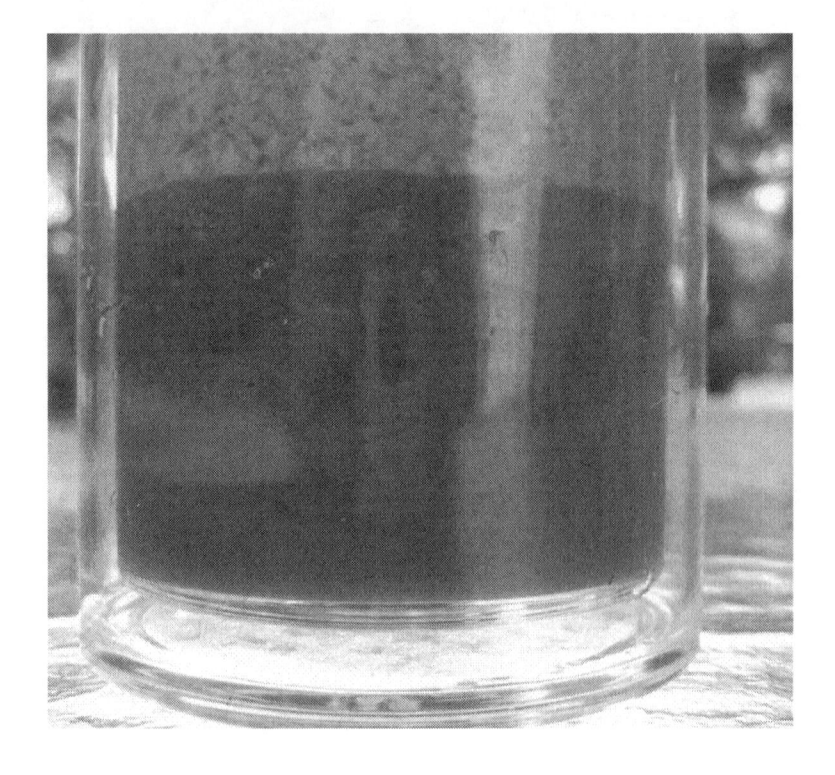

One of several versions of Tea Frappes, that the most delicious.

**Serves:** 4

**Time:** 20 mins.

**Ingredients:**

- 1 quart of water
- cups of stevia
- rind of 1 lemon
- juice of 3 lemons
- ½ cup of orange juice
- ½ cup prepared tea, strong
- 1 pineapple, finely chopped
- cups of sparkling water

**Directions:**

1 Add 1 quart of water, 2 cups of stevia, rind of 1 lemon and boil 10 minutes.

2 Strain out the lemon and cool.

3 Add juice of 3 lemons, ½ cup of orange juice, ½ cup prepared strong tea, 1 finely chopped pineapple and 2 cups of sparkling water.

4 Add more stevia if desired.

5 Freeze until granular. Enjoy!

# Sticky Buffalo Chicken Tenders

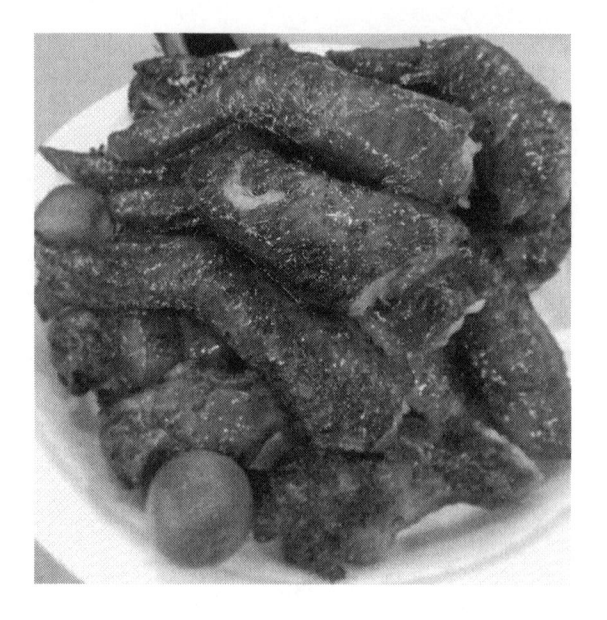

These chicken tenders be quickly become the star of any dinner party.

**Serves:** 6

**Time:** 30 mins.

**Ingredients:**

- 1lb. skinless chicken breasts, pounded into ½" thickness
- ½ cup brown stevia
- 3 tablespoons water
- 3 eggs
- ¼ cup flour
- 1/3 cup red hot sauce
- 1 cup panko bread crumbs
- ½ teaspoon garlic powder

**Directions:**

1. Set your oven to preheat to 425 degrees F. Cut the chicken breasts into strips. Add chicken to a Ziploc bag and add the flour. Shake to coat.

2. Place the bread crumbs in a bowl. Place the egg in another bowl. Dip the floured meat into the eggs then into the breadcrumbs.

3. Add chicken to a baking sheet and spray with cooking oil on top. Bake in the oven for 20 minutes.

4. Set your sauce ingredients to cook in a saucepan.

5. Toss your chicken tenders in your sauce and serve.

# Prunes in Tea Jelly

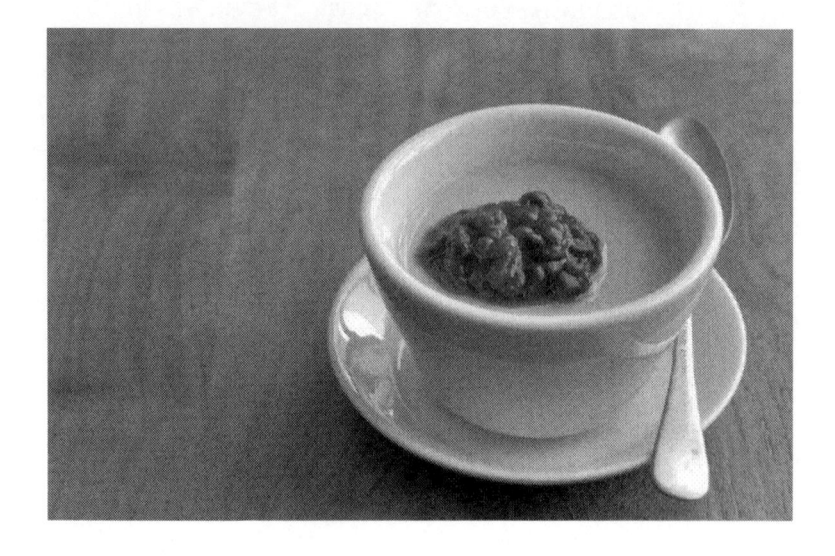

The more you like prunes, the more you will enjoy this very interesting use of tea.

**Serves:** 4

**Time:** 30 mins.

**Ingredients:**

- ½ pound prunes (with no pits)
- 1/3 cup of stevia
- 1 tablespoon of gelatin
- ¼ cup of cold water
- 4 cups prepared tea
- rind of 1 orange, grated
- 1 tablespoon candied lemon peel, finely chopped
- tablespoons lemon juice
- 1 cup of split, blanched almonds
- cream (optional)

**Directions:**

1 Cook ½ pound of prunes until tender in just enough water to cover.

2 When nearly cooked, add 1/3 cup of stevia.

3 Cool, strain and add enough tea to make 1 ½ cups.

4 Cut prunes in quarters. Soak 1 tablespoonful of gelatin in ¼ cup of cold water and dissolve in the hot prune juice and tea mixture.

5 Next add grated rind of 1 orange, 1 tablespoon of candied lemon peel, finely chopped, as well as 2 tablespoons lemon juice.

6 Set aside and stir occasionally as it thickens.

7 Then, stir in the prunes and ¼ cupful of split and blanched almonds.

8 Pour in individual molds and serve with custard or cream. Enjoy!

# Admiral Punch

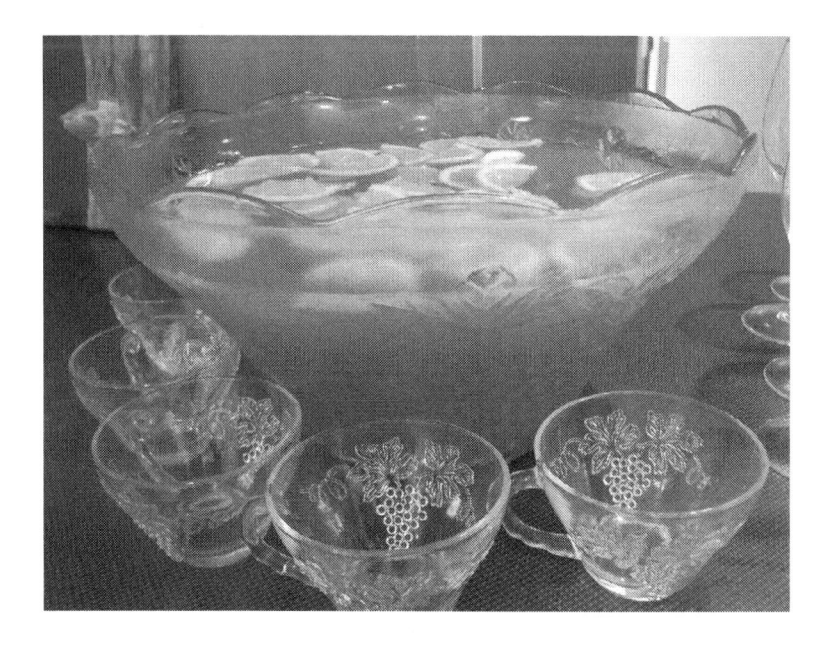

Originally, this called for a famous brand of sparkling water, but a store brand works just as well.

**Serves:** 4

**Time:** 15 mins + resting time

**Ingredients:**

- 1 quart of prepared tea
- cups of stevia
- grated rind of 1 orange
- grated rind of 3 lemons
- juice of 6 lemons
- juice of 2 oranges
- 1 cup of shredded pineapple
- 1 cup of strawberries
- bananas, sliced
- 2 cups of grape juice or ginger ale
- 1 teaspoon of almond extract
- 1 teaspoon rose water
- 1 teaspoon vanilla
- 3 quarts of sparkling water

**Directions:**

1 Pour tea into pan along with 4 cups of stevia, grated rind of 1 orange and grated rind of 3 lemons.

2 Boil for 5 minutes. Strain and let stand overnight.

3 Next day, mix together the juice of 6 lemons and 2 oranges, 1 cup of pineapple that has been shredded, 1 cup of strawberries, 3 sliced bananas, 2 cups of grape juice or ginger ale, and 1 teaspoon each of almond extract, rose water and vanilla.

4 Then, add fruit to the tea, pour into a pitcher and add ice.

5 Before serving, add 3 quarts of sparkling water.

# Scrambled Eggs with Cranberries

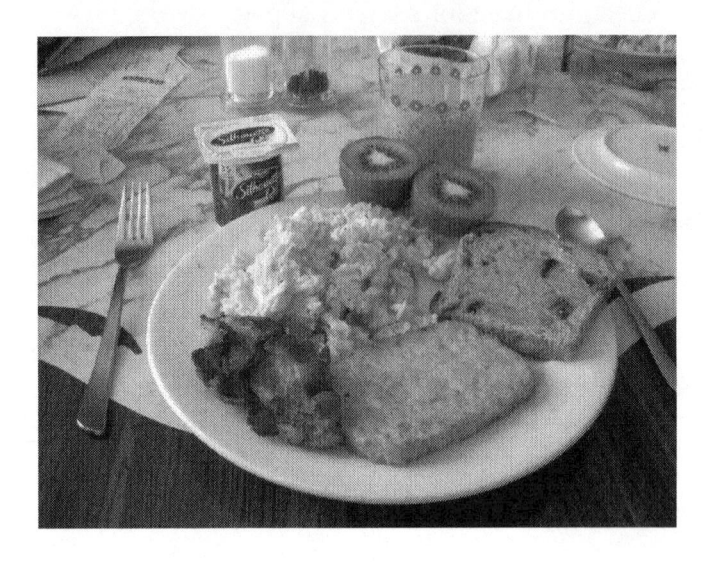

Use stevia to add a source of natural sweetness to your breakfast can add a boost of energy to the beginning of a rough day. This recipe uses cranberry for natural sweetness.

**Serves:** 2

**Time:** 10 mins

**Ingredients:**

- 4 large Eggs, beaten
- ¼ tsp Powdered Stevia
- ¼ tsp Cranberry Extract, sugar-free
- 2 tbsp Butter
- ¼ tsp Salt
- 1 tbsp Skim Milk
- 4 Cranberries

**Directions:**

1. Whisk together your eggs, stevia, cranberry extract, salt, and milk.

2. Add butter to the pressure cooker. Press BEANS/LENTILS button and melt it.

3. Pour your egg mixture then pull the eggs gently across the pot with a wooden spatula. Try not to stir constantly.

4. Cook until thickened and fully cooked (for about 2 minutes).

5. When done, turn off the cooker and transfer to a serving plate. Garnish and serve.

# Strawberry Lemon Juice

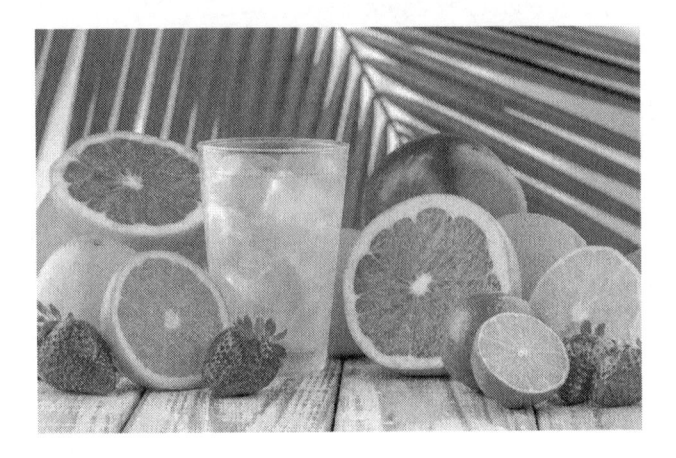

Here is another fruity drink that you are bound to enjoy.

**Time:** 5 minutes

Yield: 2 servings

**Ingredients:**

- 6 lemons, juiced
- 1 cup strawberry juice
- ½ cup raw stevia
- 3 cups water
- 1 cup ice chunks

**Directions:**

1. Combine all your ingredients in a pitcher.

2. Serve and enjoy.

# Strawberry Cheesecake Mousse

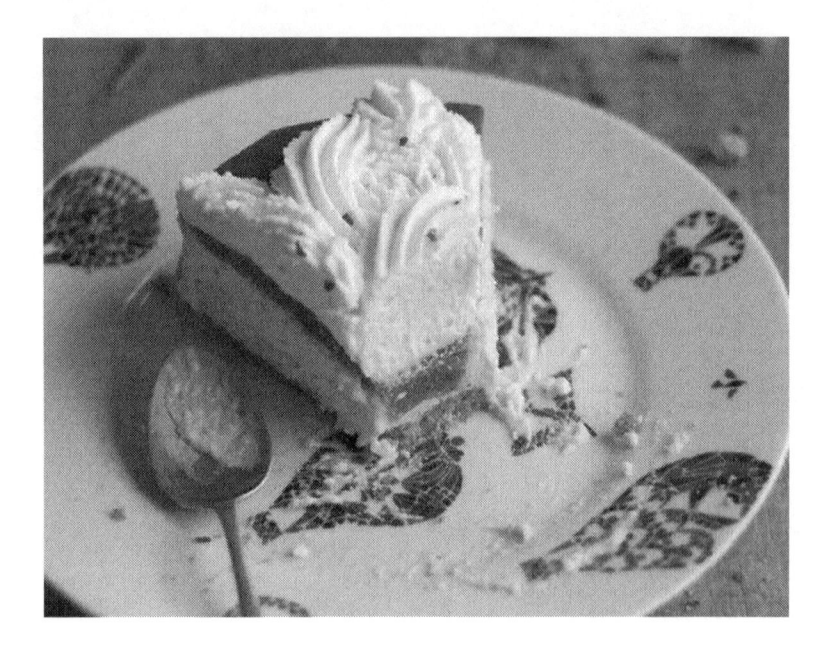

Now you can have a delicious mousse made from strawberry cheesecake filling.

**Serves:** 2

**Time:** 1 hr. 1o mins

**Ingredients:**

- 4 ounces cream cheese, room temp., crumbled
- 1 teaspoon Stevia
- 4 strawberries, sliced
- 1 tablespoon heavy cream
- 1 teaspoon vanilla extract

**Directions:**

1. Distribute your ingredients evenly in your blender. Add the cream, stevia, and vanilla. Mix together on high.

2. Toss in your strawberries then mix until combined.

3. Divide the mixture into two small dishes and set to chill for 1 hour before serving.

# Tea Julep

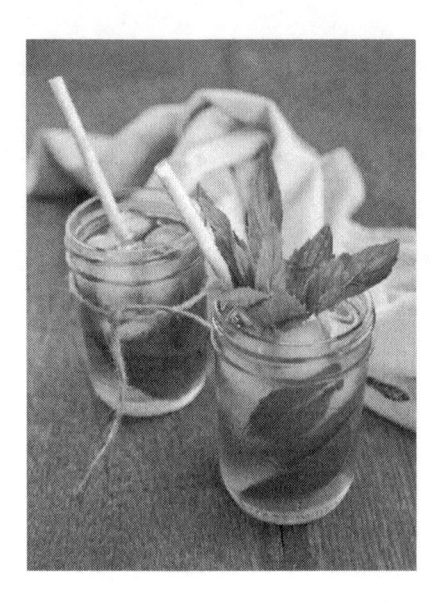

This Tea Julep is uniquely flavored and delicious.

**Serves:** 4

**Time:** 20 mins.

**Ingredients:**

- prepared tea, 1 quart
- mint, bunch
- oranges, sliced
- ½ cucumber, peeled, sliced
- 2 lemons, juiced, strained
- stevia, to taste
- 2 cups of ginger ale, chilled
- 3 strawberries, sliced

**Directions:**

1 Add your prepared tea into a large bowl then chill.

2 When cold, add in your stevia, lemon juice, cucumber, oranges and mint.

3 Set Chill for 2 hours.

4 Discard the cucumber and mint and stir in your ginger ale.

5 Garnish with fresh mint and sliced strawberries. Enjoy!

# Chia Pudding

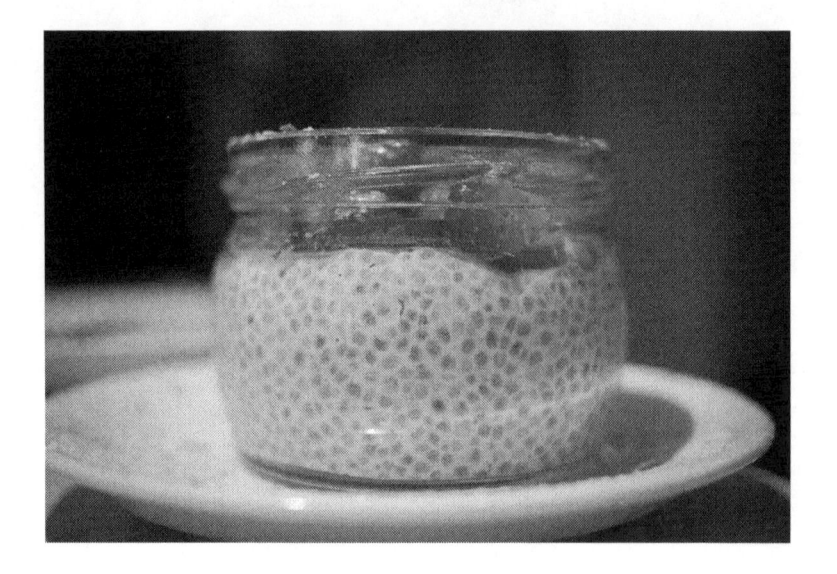

Chia has grown in popularity over the years due to its nutritional value and easiness to use. This delicious recipe is simple and can be prepped in minutes.

**Serves:** 4

**Time:** 2 hours 5 minutes

**Ingredients:**

- ½ cup chia seeds
- 2 cups almond milk
- ¼ cup almonds
- ¼ cup coconut, shredded
- 4 teaspoons stevia

**Directions:**

1. Put chia seeds in your instant pot, add coconut, almonds, stevia and milk, stir, and cover.

2. Cook on High for 3 minutes, divide into bowls and serve.

3. Enjoy!

# Apple Cheddar Waffles

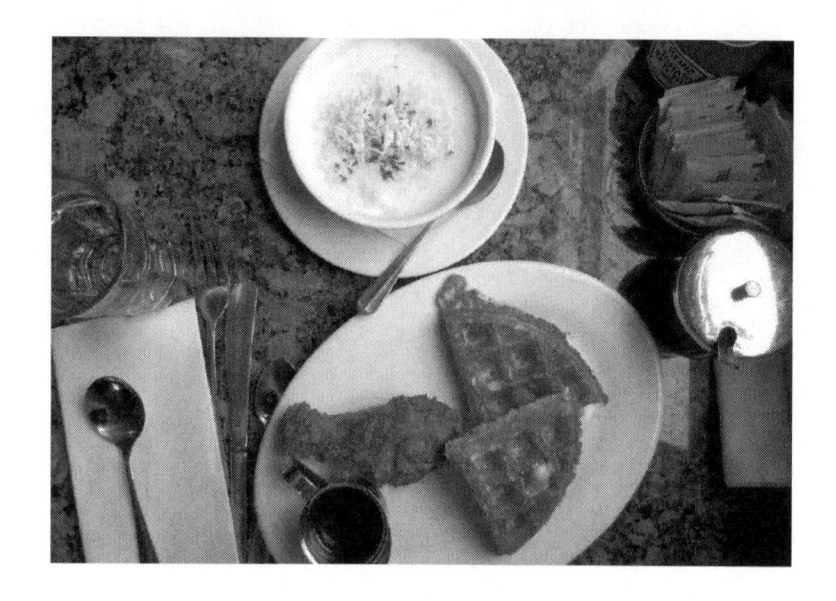

If you love cheddar cheese on apple pie, then these waffles are perfect for you.

**Serves:** 8

**Time:** 20 minutes

**Ingredients:**

- 2 cups flour
- 1 tablespoon of baking powder
- 4 tablespoons stevia
- 1 teaspoons salt
- 2 eggs, lightly whisked
- 1 cup milk
- 1/3 cup vegetable oil
- 1/2 cup shredded cheddar cheese
- 1/2 cup grated apples

**Directions:**

1. Whisk together all your dry ingredients together.

2. In a separate, small bowl, whisk all the wet ingredients together.

3. Slowly incorporate your wet ingredients with your dry, whisking constantly until smooth and lump-free.

4. Heat your waffle maker according to your manufacturer's directions. Even if you have a non-stick waffle maker, we recommend using cooking spray to prevent the cheese from sticking to the machine as it melts

5. Cook the batter according to your waffle maker's directions – every machine is slightly different regarding cooking time!

# Grape Tea Punch

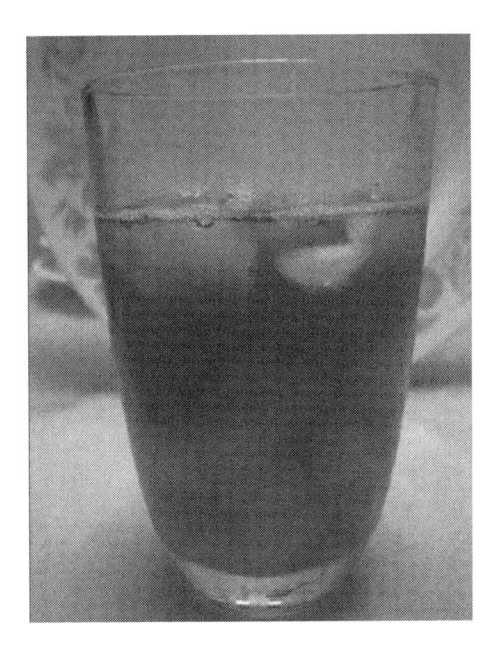

This punch is a pale purple color which is an interesting shade to achieve from any tea.

**Serves:** 12

**Time:** 20 mins.

**Ingredients:**

- 1 small pineapple, grated
- 1 cup of boiling water
- ½ cup prepared tea
- cups of water
- 2 cups of stevia
- juice of 3 oranges
- juice of 3 lemons
- 1 cup of grape juice
- 10 cups of water

**Directions:**

1 Grate 1 small pineapple. To each cup of pineapple, add 1 cup of boiling water and simmer 10 minutes.

2 Make a syrup by boiling 2 cups of water and 2 cups of stevia for 10 minutes. Add ½ cup hot tea to the syrup and set aside until cool.

3 Then, add the strained juice of 3 oranges and 3 lemons as well as 1 cup of grape juice and 10 cups of water. Enjoy!

# Mug Birthday Cake

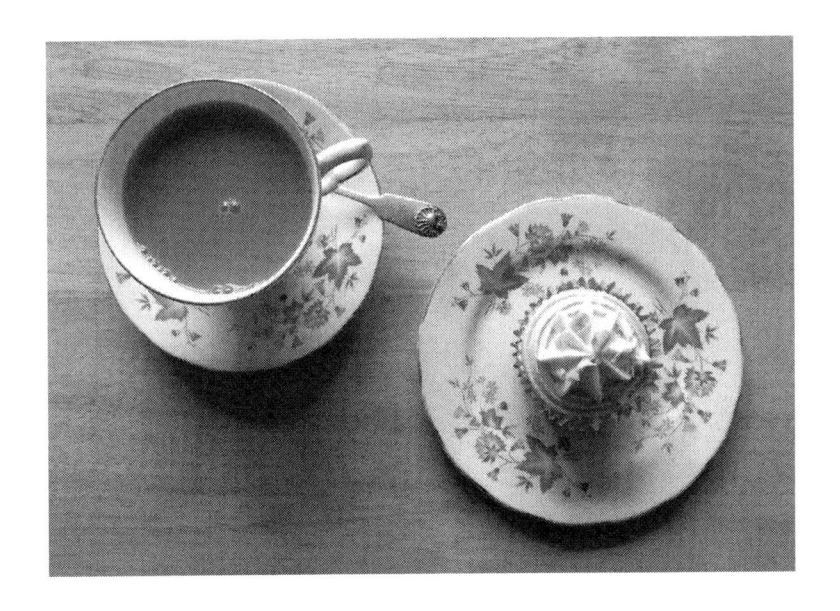

Celebrate your beloved birthday with this tasty and sweet Birthday Cake in a Mug.

**Serves:** 8

**Time:** 5 mins.

**Ingredients:**

- Funfetti cake mix (1 box)
- Instant pudding mix (1, vanilla flavor)

**Glaze Ingredients:**

- Stevia (1/3 cup, powdered)
- Cocoa powder (1 ½ tsp)
- Egg white (1)
- Oil (1 tbsp)
- Water (1 tbsp)

**Directions:**

1. Using cooking spray, lightly grease a large coffee mug then empty the cake mix into the mug.

2. Next, add the egg white, oil, and water. Blend with a fork until smooth.

3. Microwave on high for approximately 2 minutes.

4. While the cake is cooking, add 1 ½ teaspoon of water to other glaze ingredients in a sandwich bag. Seal the sandwich bag and knead until the glaze is smooth.

5. When done, remove from the microwave and cut a small hole in the corner of the sandwich bag.

6. Squeeze the glaze onto the cake. Enjoy warm.

# June Plum Drink

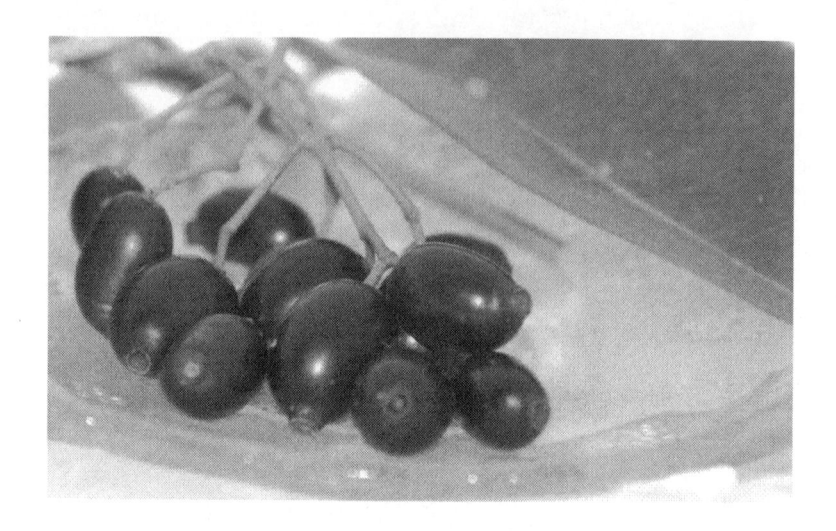

This drink is tangy, rich in vitamin C and serves as a refreshing summer drink.

**Serves:** 6

**Time:** 15 minutes

**Ingredients:**

- 6 whole June Plum
- 1 oz. root ginger
- 8 tbsp. raw stevia
- 4 cups water

**Directions:**

1. Wash June plum thoroughly.

2. Dice and remove seed.

3. Wash ginger properly, chop or grate ginger.

4. Add your ingredients into a blender then run until smooth.

5. Strain and adjust to desired taste.

6. Serve with crushed or cubed ice.

# Yellow Bird Stevia Cocktail

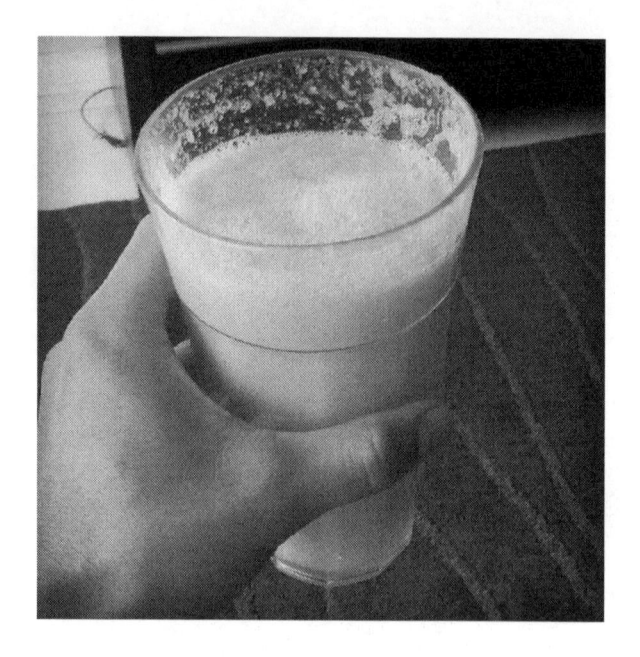

A refreshing stevia free cocktail.

**Serves:** 2

**Time:** 15 minutes

**Ingredients:**

- 1 oz. lime juice
- ½ oz. raw stevia syrup
- 6 oz. orange juice
- ½ oz. Tia Maria
- 2 oz. over proof rum
- ½ oz. crème de banana
- 6 oz. Galliano liqueur

**Directions:**

1. Blend or shake ingredients together with ice cubes

2. Serve in a 12oz. glass, nicely garnished.

# Chocolate Berry Cheesecake

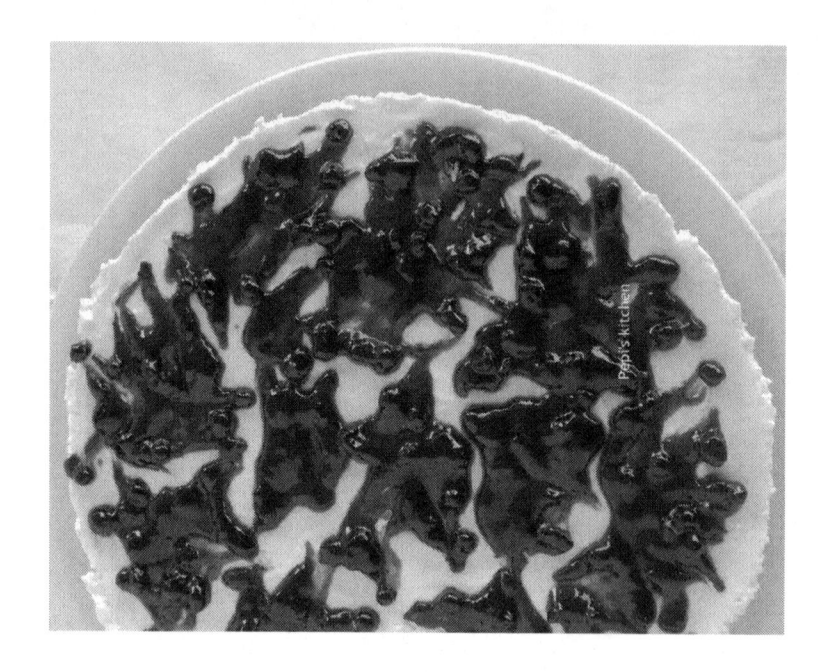

Finally, an easy dessert that can be pushed in the oven and ready in minutes.

**Serves:** 16

**Time:** 35 minutes

**Ingredients:**

- 4 tablespoon butter, melted
- 1 ½ cup chocolate cookie, crumbed
- 3 packages low-fat cream cheese
- 2 tablespoon cornstarch
- 1 cup stevia
- 3 large eggs
- ½ cup plain Greek yogurt
- 1 tablespoon vanilla extract
- 4-ounce milk chocolate
- 4-ounce white chocolate
- 4-ounce bittersweet chocolate
- 1 cup stevia- covered cranberries

**Directions:**

1. Brush ramekins or a spring form pan with oil. Set aside.

2. Make the crust by combining butter with cookie crumbs. Press the dough at the bottom of the pan. Place in the freezer to set.

3. Beat cream cheese in your mixer on low speed until smooth.

4. Add cornstarch and stevia and continue mixing until well combined.

5. Add an egg at a time while mixing. Scrape the sides of the bowl as needed.

6. Add in your vanilla and yogurt then mix until well combined. Divide the batter in three bowls. Set aside.

7. Melt the milk chocolate in the microwave oven for 30 seconds twice until completely melted.

8. Whisk the chocolate into one of the bowls of the cheesecake batter. Do the same thing with the white and bittersweet chocolates.

9. Take the spring form pan out from the fridge. Pour the dark chocolate batter as the first layer, followed by the white chocolate and milk chocolate.

10. Put aluminum foil on top of the spring form pan. Pour water on the Instant Pot and place the steamer rack. Place the spring form pan and close the lid.

11. Cook on high for 10 minutes. Do a natural pressure release to open the lid.

12. Take the cheesecake out and refrigerate for 1 hour.

13. Serve with stevia-covered cranberries.

# Zucchini and Carrot Noodles with Tomato Sauce

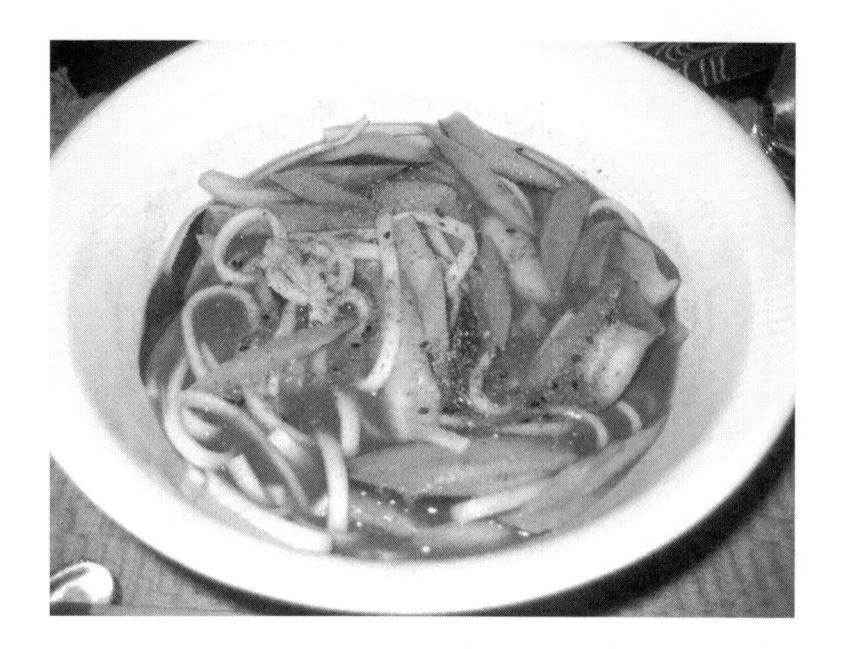

A colourful tasty dish with delicious flavours and vitamins entrapped.

**Serving size:** 2

**Overall Time:** 20 mins.

**Ingredients:**

- 2 zucchinis, julienne
- 2 carrots, peeled, julienne
- 1 cup tomatoes, chopped
- 2 tablespoon stevia
- ¼ pinch salt
- ¼ cup sun dried tomatoes
- ½ cup cream
- ½ cup water

**Directions:**

1. To create zucchini noodles (zoodles) using a vegetable peeler, shave the zucchini with the peeler lengthwise until you get to the core with the seeds.

2. Turn the zucchini, and repeat the process is creating long strips. Continue repeating the process until you have shaved all the zucchini into strips and discard the seeds.

3. Now lay your strips on a cutting board, and slice lengthwise to the desired thickness that you would like your zoodle to be.

4. In a pressure cooker add water, tomatoes, sun dried tomatoes, stevia, salt and mix well.

5. Let it cook for 4 minutes and close the lid. Add in cream and mix, transfer to a blender and blend well. In platter add carrot and zucchini zoodles and top with tomato sauce.

6. Enjoy.

# Simple Tapioca Pudding

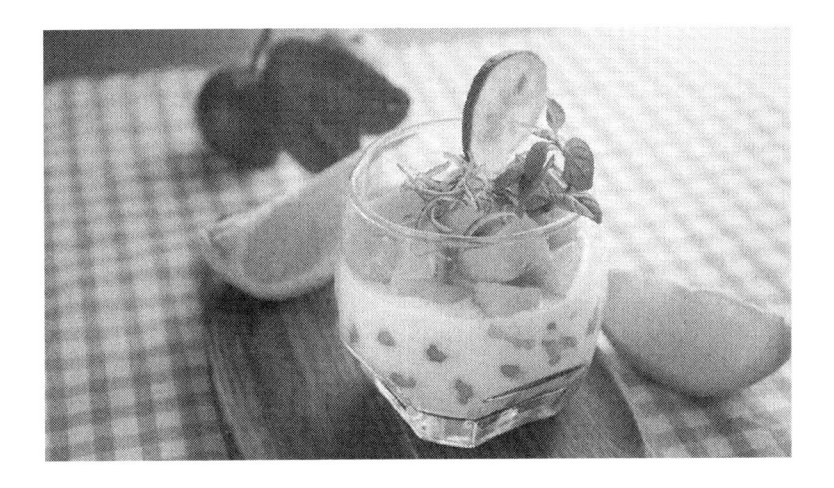

Tapioca is literally the new Chia. This recipe will blow your mind if you have never tasted Tapioca pudding.

**Serves:** 4

**Time:** 20 minutes

**Ingredients:**

- 1 and ½ cups water
- 1/3 cup tapioca pearls
- 2 tablespoons stevia
- 1 and ¼ cup low-fat milk
- Zest of ½ lemon, grated

**Directions:**

1. Put tapioca in a heatproof bowl, add milk, ½ cup water, lemon zest and stevia and toss.

2. Add the water to your instant pot, add the steamer basket, add the bowl inside and cover.

3. Cook on High for 10 minutes, divide into bowls and serve.

4. Enjoy!

# Delicious Banana Nut Oatmeal

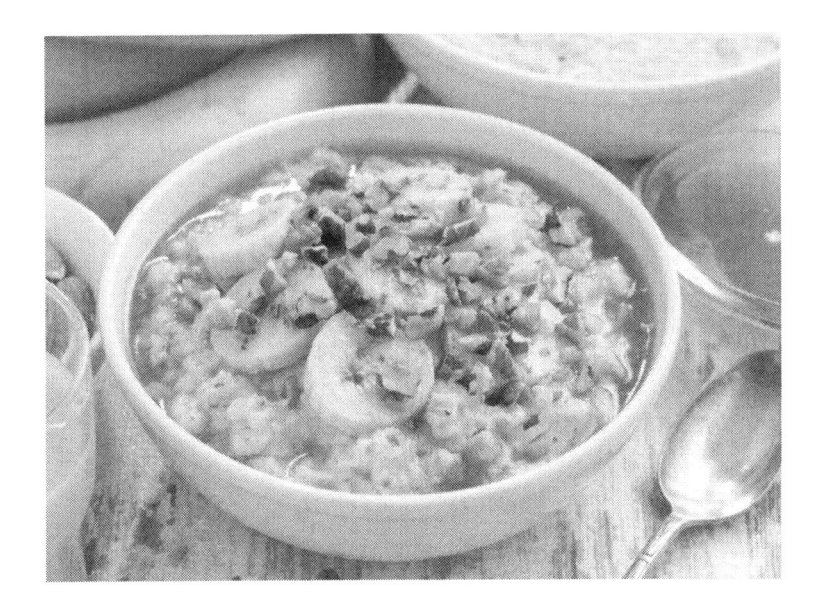

Here is another delicious oatmeal that will make your mornings even better.

**Serves:** 3

**Time:** 25 Minutes

**Ingredients:**

- 2 Bananas, sliced
- 3 cups water
- 1 cup steel cut oats
- 1 teaspoon cinnamon
- ½ cup almonds, sliced
- 1 teaspoon stevia

**Directions:**

1. In an instant pot, stir together one banana, water, oats, and cinnamon. Seal the lid then switch to manual for 15 minutes.

2. When done, natural release pressure for about 10 minutes and then open the lid.

3. Transfer the oatmeal into a serving bowl and stir in stevia, almond slices and the remaining banana.

# Tea Ice Cream

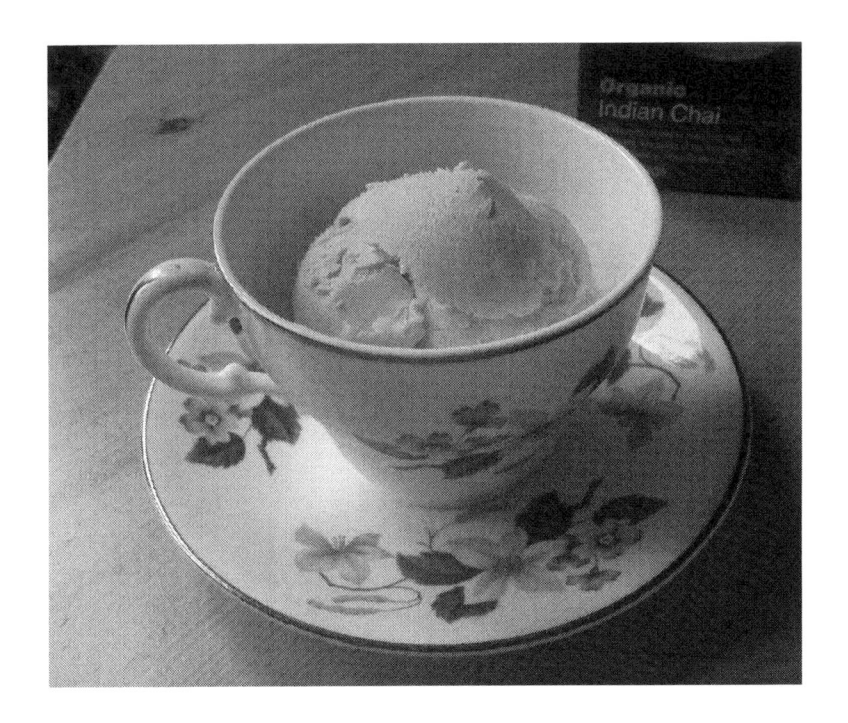

This tea based ice cream is easy and good.

**Serves:** 4

**Time:** 30 mins.

**Ingredients:**

- 1 cup of prepared tea, strong (herbal or flavored tea work best)
- tablespoons of stevia
- cups of vanilla custard
- 1 tablespoon heavy cream

**Directions:**

1 Add 4 tablespoons of stevia to 1 cup of very strong tea.

2 When cool, mix with 2 cups of vanilla custard and 1 tablespoon heavy cream.

3 Freeze. Enjoy when set.

# Rum Punch

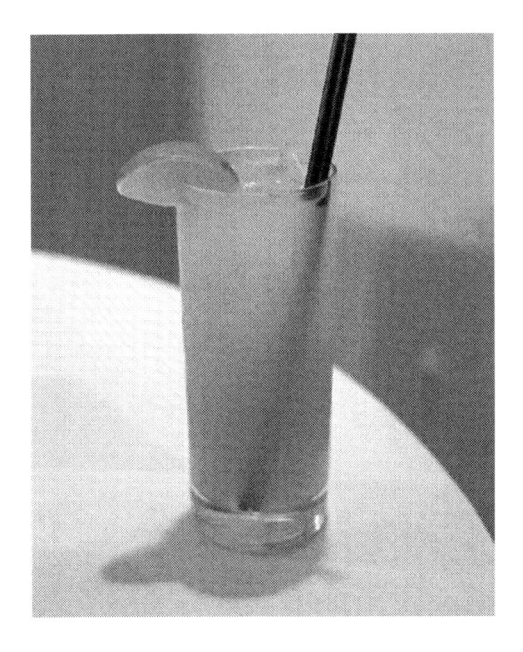

Here is a delicious punch great for adult events.

**Serves:** 10

**Time:** 15 minutes

**Ingredients:**

- 4 fl. oz. lemon juice
- 8 fl. oz. strawberry juice (unsweetened)
- 5 tbsp. raw stevia
- 12 fl. oz. fruit juice (a combination of orange and pineapple juice)
- 1 pt. over proof white rum

**Directions:**

1. Combine all ingredients in a punch bowl.

2. Adjust to desired taste.

3. Garnish with slices of lime or pineapple.

4. Refrigerate, and serve over ice.

# Mug Banana Bread

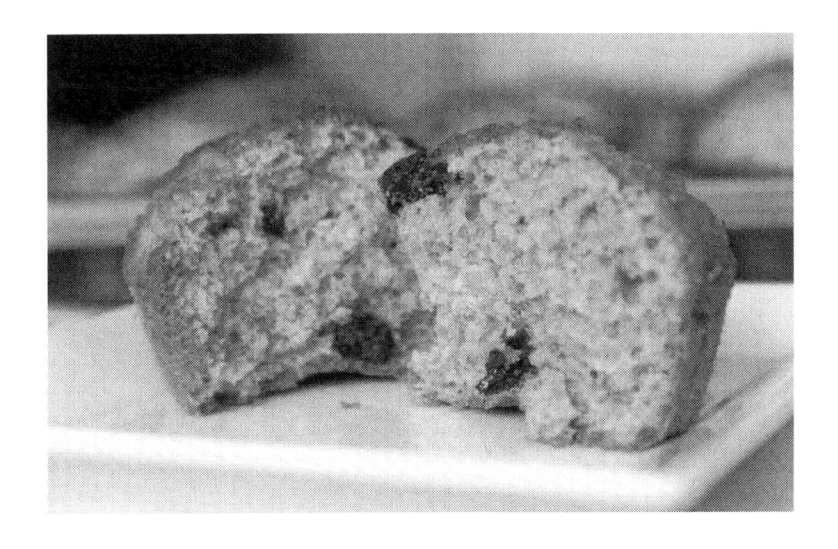

Enjoy this sweet, delicious Banana Bread in a mug.

**Serves:** 4

**Time:** 5 mins

**Ingredients:**

- 1 oven proof mug
- Flour (1/4 cup, all-purpose)
- Stevia (2 tbsp, granulated)
- Baking soda (1/4 tsp)
- Cinnamon (1/8 tsp, ground)
- pinch of salt
- Walnuts (1 tbsp, finely chopped)
- Chocolate chips (2 tbsp, mini)
- Banana (1/2, ripe)
- Egg (1)
- Canola or vegetable oil (1 tbsp)

**Directions:**

1. Preheat your oven to 350 degrees Fahrenheit.

2. Combine the flour, stevia, cinnamon, baking soda, salt, walnuts, and 1 tablespoon chocolate chips. Set aside.

3. Mash the banana, egg and oil in a small bowl to combine with fork.

4. Combine the wet and dry ingredients and pour into an oven safe mug.

5. Bake until done (about 25-30 minutes).

# Instant Pot Blueberry Oatmeal

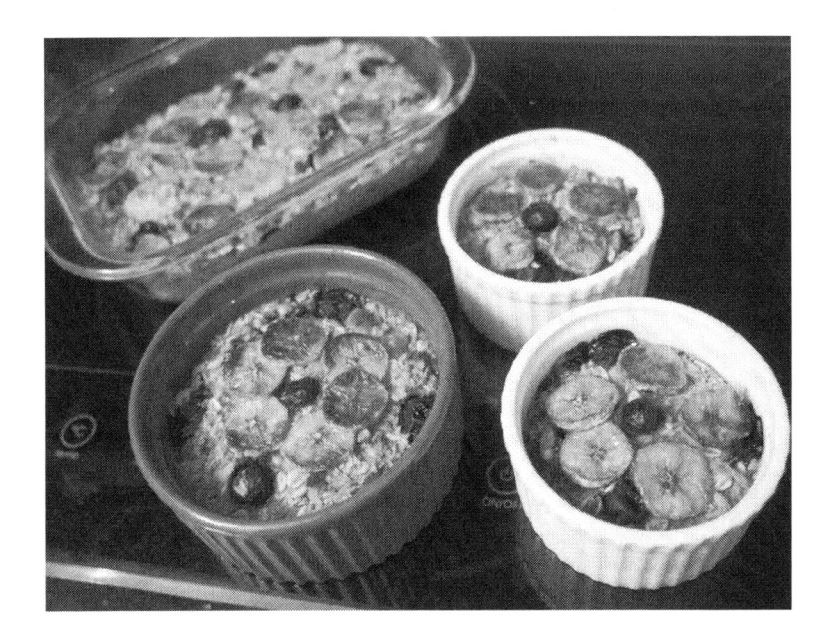

Add a dash of fruit to your next morning oatmeal using this easy recipe.

**Serves:** 6

**Time:** 20 Minutes

**Ingredients:**

- 1 cup blueberries
- 2 cups coconut milk
- 1/2 cup stevia
- 2 1/4 cups whole oats
- 1/4 cup almond flour blend
- 3 cups water
- 1/8 teaspoon salt
- 1 teaspoon vanilla

**Directions:**

1. Add all your ingredients into your instant pot then cook for 15 minutes on high pressure. Serve warm.

# Avocado Salsa Zoodles

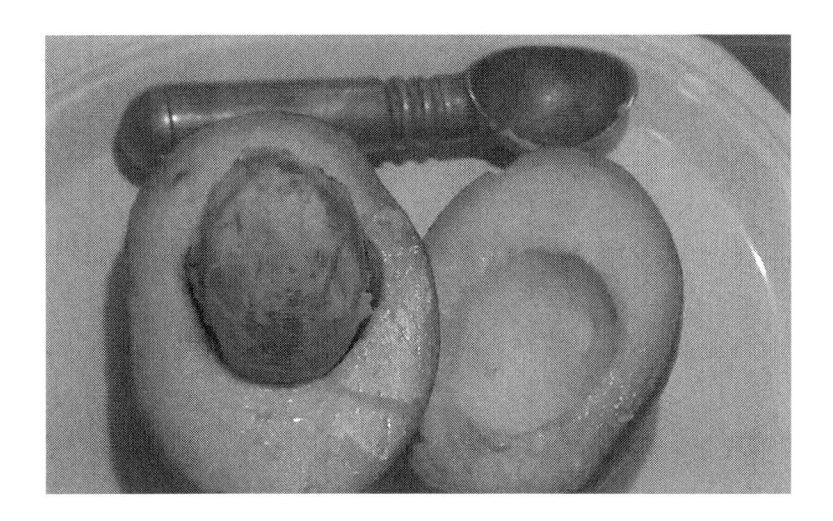

The avocado in this recipe serves as a creamy compliment to the zoodles of this recipe to form a filling low carb pasta dish.

**Serving size:** 2

**Overall Time:** 20 mins.

**Ingredients:**

- 2 medium zucchinis
- 1 Hass avocado, pitted, chunks
- ¼ teaspoon salt
- ¼ teaspoon black pepper
- 4 tablespoons lemon juice
- 2 tablespoon apple cider vinegar
- 3 tablespoon stevia
- ½ teaspoon dill, chopped
- Few coriander leaves for garnishing

**Directions:**

1. To create zucchini noodles (zoodles) using a vegetable peeler, shave the zucchini with the peeler lengthwise until you get to the core with the seeds. Turn the zucchini, and repeat the process is creating long strips.

2. Continue repeating the process until you have shaved all the zucchini into strips and discard the seeds.

3. Now lay your strips on a cutting board, and slice lengthwise to the desired thickness that you would like your zoodle to be.

4. Transfer zoodles into your slow cooker, close the lid, and cook for 5 minutes. Combine avocado, dill, salt, pepper, stevia, vinegar, lemon juice, and mix.

5. Place zoodle in serving platter and top with mango salsa. Garnish with coriander leaves. Serve and enjoy.

# Conclusion

Thank you for allowing me to take you along this sugar free journey with me in the Zero Sugar Stevia Cookbook. I hope you enjoyed all 30 stevia recipes that were featured in this book and that you were able to pinpoint a new favorite meal.

If you wouldn't mind taking a few minutes to leave a positive review on the platform on which you purchased the book, that would be amazing.

Cheers!

# About the Author

Born in New Germantown, Pennsylvania, Stephanie Sharp received a Masters degree from Penn State in English Literature. Driven by her passion to create culinary masterpieces, she applied and was accepted to The International Culinary School of the Art Institute where she excelled in French cuisine. She has married her cooking skills with an aptitude for business by opening her own small cooking school where she teaches students of all ages.

Stephanie's talents extend to being an author as well and she has written over 400 e-books on the art of cooking and baking that include her most popular recipes.

Sharp has been fortunate enough to raise a family near her hometown in Pennsylvania where she, her husband and children live in a beautiful rustic house on an extensive piece of land. Her other passion is taking care of the furry members of her family which include 3 cats, 2 dogs and a potbelly pig named Wilbur.

Watch for more amazing books by Stephanie Sharp coming out in the next few months.

# Author's Afterthoughts

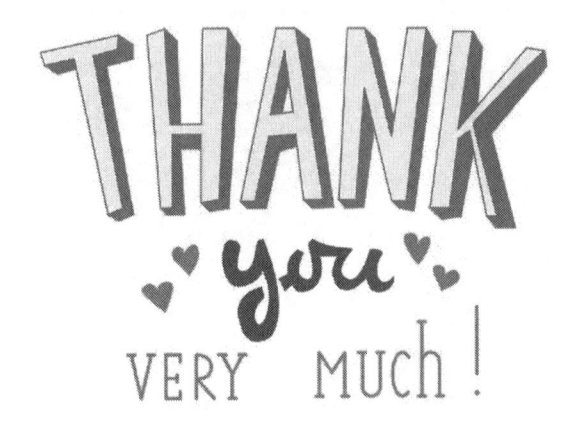

I am truly grateful to you for taking the time to read my book. I cherish all of my readers! Thanks ever so much to each of my cherished readers for investing the time to read this book!

With so many options available to you, your choice to buy my book is an honour, so my heartfelt thanks at reading it from beginning to end!

I value your feedback, so please take a moment to submit an honest and open review on Amazon so I can get valuable insight into my readers' opinions and others can benefit from your experience.

*Thank you for taking the time to review!*

**Stephanie Sharp**

*For announcements about new releases, please follow my author page on Amazon.com!*

*You can find that at:*

*https://www.amazon.com/author/stephanie-sharp*

*or Scan **QR-code** below.*

Made in the USA
Columbia, SC
03 July 2021